AF882732

Rise:

Substance Abuse Treatment Program

A Poly-Therapeutic Substance Abuse Treatment Workbook

Written by Justin Nutt, LSCSW, LCSW

Product of Nurstead Consulting Services

Note to Participants

INTRODUCTION:

First, we want to say congratulations for taking the first step to healing and creating a new future. Over the next several weeks, you will have many more reasons to celebrate, but those successes will come with difficulties, as well. These difficulties will not be anything that you are incapable of overcoming; they will simply be uncomfortable points which can be stepping stones to growth. Any true growth or change comes as the result of the willingness to look within and see the negative as well as the positive. No one can force you to look within with clarity, and no one can force you to be honest, but if you aren't willing to be honest with yourself, no change can or will occur.

THE PROCESS:

The process of each group will be similar. A check-in process will occur to discuss any changes since the last session and to offer help as needed. After the check-in process, or as part of it, depending on your group leader's style, a review of homework will occur. This is for one main reason: the beauty of group work is the fact members often learn more and create more change as a result of their interactions rather than as a result of the lecture component of group work. While more is learned from the interactions and discussions between members, the group leader serves to provide the needed information that assists with the worksheets and discussions. It is important to participate in the discussions that occur, but also to be respectful and listen to the thoughts of others. Avoidance of either will hinder you from getting the maximum out of each session and the program itself.

WORKSHEETS:

Each week there will be a worksheet to be completed as part of the learning process This homework should be completed honestly. It is not something on which you will be judged; it is for you and your growth. Each worksheet has been specially created based on a evidence-based theories of substance abuse and clinical treatment to address a specific aspect of the change and recovery process. These worksheets will be used as a part of the check-in and group discussion process.

REMEMBER:

It is important to be involved, be honest, and be willing to learn from others and yourself. Learning is not a matter of judging the difference; judging creates stones that weigh us down, but learning creates stones that raise us up.

Introduction to Rise and Cognitive Distortions

SESSION 1:

Group Rules, Norms, and Expectations

- Group safety: No violence or threats towards staff or other group members is allowed.
- Confidentiality: It is important that whatever is said in the group is kept within the group.
- Respect: It is important that each member of the group be respected. While you may not agree with other members' beliefs, they are still worthy of respect, just as you are.
- Participation: Some members may be more comfortable sharing than others, but for the group process to work, all participants need to participate.
- Absences and Tardiness: For the group process to work, it is important that each group member be here on time. If a member misses more than **TWO** sessions, that member will be asked to not attend the group anymore.

Cognitive Distortions

Cognitive distortions, or thinking traps, are ways of thinking that prevent us from logical thought about people, places, things, and events. Identification of which mistakes of thought are present is the best way to start to create change connected to our thinking patterns. Below is an index of different cognitive distortions. This is not a complete list, but many of the most common cognitive distortions are defined below. It is also important to remember that at times the distortions in our thinking can include more than one or a combination of cognitive distortions about the same item.

Overgeneralization: Allowing one or two events to be taken as proof of how someone or something thinks or acts. Overgeneralizing happens when there is the belief that something always happens or never happens.

Filtering: Extracting the good or bad of an event to focus on the negative and ignore the positive or vice versa.

Magnifying: Taking a small piece of an interaction or characteristic of a person and making it larger than it truly is. Things are blown out of proportion, and a molehill is made into a mountain.

Minimizing: Deeming a large issue to be unimportant and unworthy of focus (the opposite of magnifying).

Catastrophizing: Seeing any unpleasant occurrence as the worst possible outcome. An event may not have even happened and the expectation of how terrible it was or will be is already being considered.

Black and White Thinking: Viewing something as all or nothing. It is either good or bad; there exists no in-between. When this distortion is present, there is the lack of understanding that most times people, places, things, and events are made up of many aspects - both good and bad, right and wrong.

Blaming: Accusing another person completely for negative events occurring. Rather than accepting we did something to impact an event, our faults, failures, and other negative aspects are believed to be someone else's fault.

Personalization: Placing all the blame of something on oneself as if one had the ability to control the event entirely (opposite of blaming).

Emotional Reasoning: Removing logical aspects and focusing solely on the emotional; as a result, the person's emotions are taken as fact. An example would be "If I am scared, then there is real danger."

Mindreading: Believing one knows exactly what another person is thinking. It is mindreading that causes us to believe we know why another person did what he or she did.

Fortunetelling: Believing one knows what is going to happen before it happens. This distortion often leads the person to act in a manner which in turn creates a negative outcome.

Homework

Craving Levels:

S ___ M ___ T ___ W ___ T ___ F ___ S ___

What cognitive distortions are common in your thinking?

1. ____
2. ____
3. ____

<u>For each of these cognitive distortions, work through the following steps:</u>

Cognitive distortion: ____________________________

Distorted thought: ____

Exception that disproves thought: ______________________________

Factual thought: ____

How would events turn out differently without distortion?

____

Cognitive distortion: ____________________________

Distorted thought: ____

Exception that disproves thought: ______________________________

Factual thought: ____

How would events turn out differently without distortion?

____

Cognitive distortion: ________________________________

Distorted thought: ____

____

Exception that disproves thought: ____

____

Factual thought: ____

____

How would events turn out differently without distortion?

____

____

The ABC's of CBT

SESSION 2:

ABCDEF Model of CBT

Creating change requires the ability to not only identify the cognitive distortions that exist, but also to dispute these cognitive distortions to create different outcomes. A is the activating event; this is what happens, and is an item generally not within our control. B is our belief about the event; this is where the cognitive distortions come into play. C is the consequences of our beliefs about the event; this is the outcome that is the result of our thoughts and feelings about what happened. A and C are items we can't directly change, but it is disputing the beliefs that creates change. D stands for disputing these beliefs. E is the effective new belief created through the act of disputing the cognitive distortions. Lastly, F is the fitting consequence of the activating event.

Just as consequences (C) are a natural response to our beliefs (B) and the activating event (A), the fitting consequences (F) are a natural result of the new effective beliefs (E). By learning to look at our beliefs and having a willingness to dispute the mistaken beliefs we hold, we are able to create a new and lasting belief which changes the way we react.

Example

A	activating event	My girlfriend/boyfriend treats me poorly for being late to our date.
B	belief about event	I deserve this. I am not good enough. No one likes me. I can never do anything right.
C	consequences	Blaming myself for the accident and being late, I go out and drink, become angry, then yell and scream.
D	disputing evidence	I was late because there was an accident on the highway which caused traffic.
E	effective new belief	I am not a terrible person because something out of my control made me late.
F	fitting consequence	Discussion with girlfriend/boyfriend about how I feel leads to understanding that her/his anger is not about my actions.

Homework

Craving Levels:

S ___ M ___ T ___ W ___ T ___ F ___ S ___

Activating event			
Belief about the events, thoughts, and emotions			
Consequences of beliefs and emotions			
Disputing evidence of these thoughts			
Effective new belief about the event			
Fitting consequences as a result of effective beliefs			

Creating Flowing Change

SESSION 3:

Flowchart of Dialectical Thinking

In computer programming, as a program is being designed, the programmer creates a flow chart to show the processes that are a part of the program before the coding begins. This model is a great way to show the process of change in thinking patterns from emotion based to logic based.

START in this process is the permanent starting point, that is to say, it is merely who we are. While this impacts and clouds our thinking, it is not part of the emotional or the logical path, but is our world view.

Next comes the input, or the event that triggers the start of our thinking "program." This is something we generally do not control by itself, and as such, no change occurs at this point.

Next is the symbol for process, the emotional thought – our feelings and beliefs. If you continue on without stopping to think about the more logical side of an event, you make a decision based on emotions alone, and the thoughts, feelings, and beliefs, along with the decision we place on the event, create the reaction, and as a result, lead to the outcome, which is often negative because it is not based on all the facts.

When working to create change, you learn to pause earlier and earlier in the process until you get to a point where you may have the emotional thought, but you also immediately have the logical thought, as well. The logical side follows the same process as the emotional, but the decision, reaction, and outcome cycle is vastly different most times because it includes not only your emotions, but logical thoughts about the event, as well.

Homework

Craving Levels:

S ___ M ___ T ___ W ___ T ___ F ___ S ___

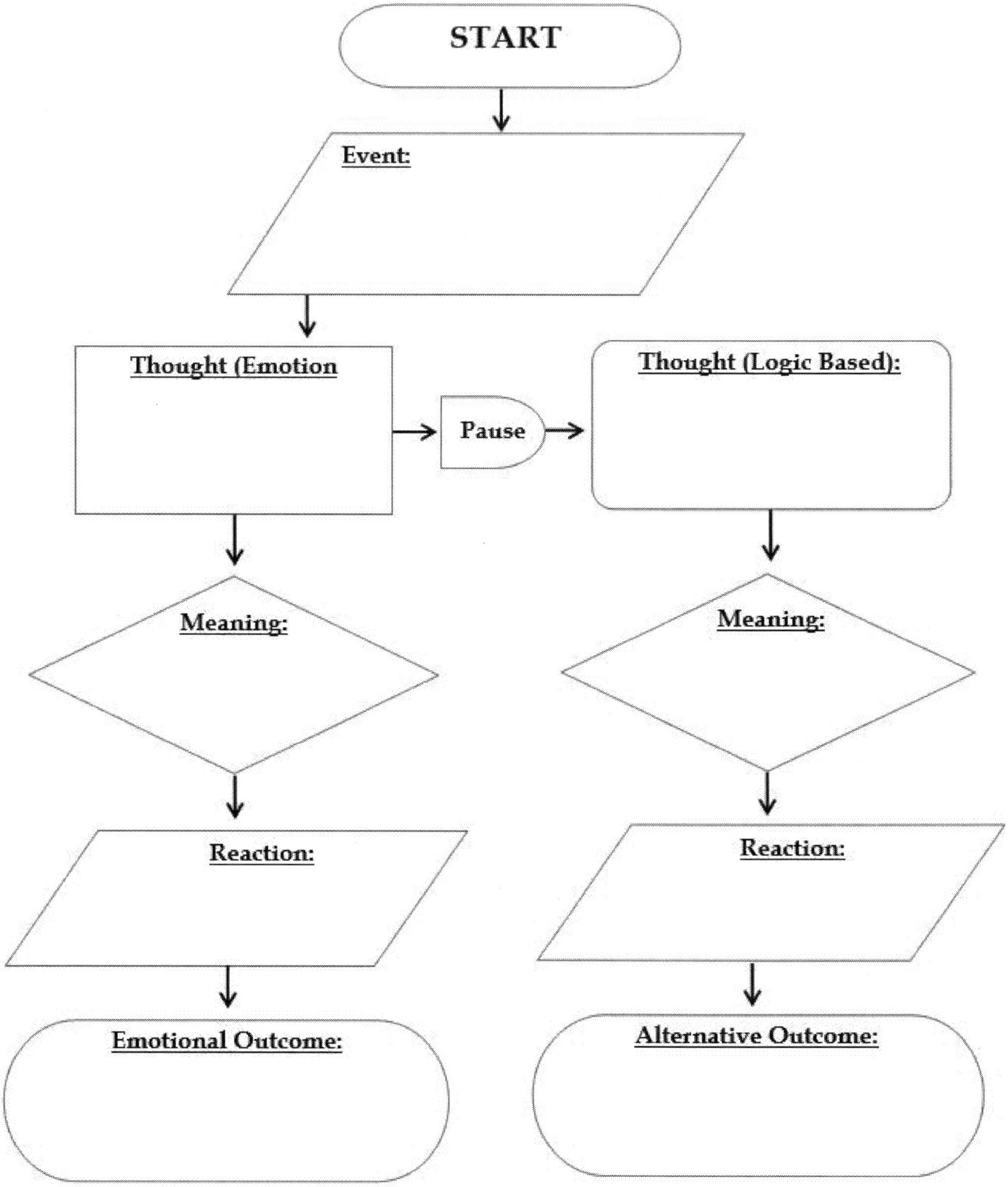

Recovery and the Stages of Change

SESSION 4:

Stages of Change

Pre-contemplation: This is a stage that precedes change. During the pre-contemplation phase, a person may realize there are negative outcomes to his or her behavior, but doesn't believe the behavior is problematic, so there is no need to change. At this stage alcoholics or addicts often believe that those around them are the ones with a problem.

Contemplation: This is the stage where change truly begins. During the contemplation phase, a person begins to question if he or she has a problem and needs to make changes. At this stage, there is commonly a large amount of back and forth between believing help and change is needed and the rejection of this idea.

Preparation: This stage is the point when a person begins to prepare to take action. During the preparation phase, an individual has accepted responsibility for his or her actions and understands that change needs to occur. It is at this point one begins to gather information or seek referrals for help. A person may also set a timeline for his or her treatment.

Action: This is the stage where the work is done. It is during the action phase that individuals enter into treatment, be it AA, residential programs, or outpatient therapy. At this stage there is an emotional, mental, and spiritual engagement in the change process. New skills and understanding are gained and put into use to create a shift in addiction-related behavior and create sobriety and recovery.

Maintenance: This is the stage where a person has made adjustments to his or her behavior and patterns of thinking, thus gaining an understanding of self and actions. These skills have become a part of one's behavior, and they are utilized to create a new routine. It is during the maintenance phase that most people leave residential treatment and return to their everyday lives.

Relapse: This is a return to substance use, and it often occurs as a part of recovery. Unlike the other stages, relapse can happen at any point during the process. It can happen during preparation, action, and maintenance. No matter where relapse occurs, an individual returns back to pre-contemplation, but most generally once the substances are out of a person's system, he or she quickly returns to the action stage and subsequently to maintenance with additional understanding resulting from relapse.

Homework

Craving Levels:

S ___ M ___ T ___ W ___ T ___ F ___ S ___

Stage 1 Pre-contemplation: Believing there is no problem with behavior or need to change.	
Stage 2 Contemplation: Recognizing a problem exists and considering change.	
Stage 3 Preparation: Accepting responsibility and gathering information.	
Stage 4 Action: Entering treatment; attending self-help groups; engaging mentally and emotionally.	
Stage 5 Maintenance: Adjusting to new behaviors; using skills to sustain change.	
Stage 6 Relapse: Returning to the use of drugs and/or alcohol.	

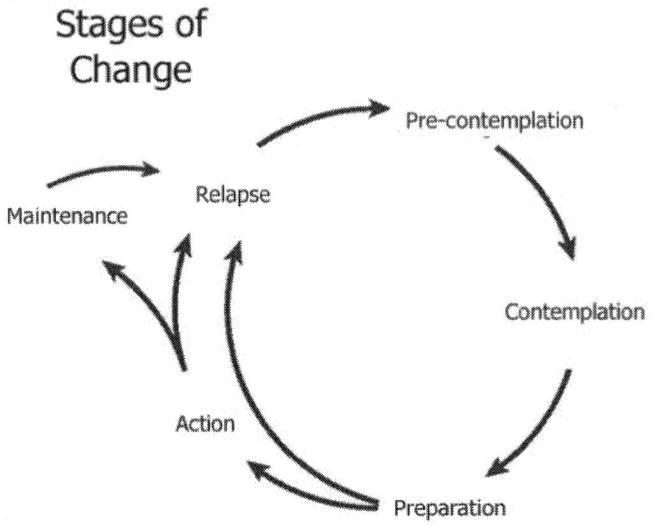

In what stage do you feel you are currently? ______________________________

What makes you believe that to be your stage? ______________________________

____

____

What thoughts do you have about your current stage? ______________________________

____

____

What will help you reach the next stage? ______________________________

____

____

Use Recall Protection

SESSION 5:

Mental Cues

Mental cues are connected to those internal thoughts, but they are not about our internal message. They are about the way we think about substance use. Mental cues can be widespread in nature, ranging from what items are being kept secret or not being talked about to thinking that drinking or drug use is the answer to a problem. Preceding relapse, often there is the glamorizing or euphoric remembrance of the times when a person drank or used drugs. Fantasizing is another often occurring mental cue that, if left unchecked, commonly leads to relapse.

Physical Cues

Physical cues are indicators of an urge or craving to use based on internal and autonomic reactions, that is to say, items which happen without our awareness or control. Common cues attached to urges and a desire to use are things like a change in breathing, increased heart rate, feeling flush or cool; all of these are cues. Cues are something that are very individual, so while two people may have shared cues, rarely will they share all of the same cues connected to every situation. For some people, when they are angry their ears turn red; for others, breathing may increase, and still others may have some sort of an eye twitch. All of these are physical cues. Another thing to remember is that the same cue can be connected to different emotions for different people or can be connected to several emotions for the same person. A good example of this is someone's face turning red. Is it the result of anger, embarrassment, amusement? Recognizing your physical cues can help an individual also recognize precursors to potential relapse.

Behavioral Cues

Behavioral cues are often confused with physical cues but are exactly what they sound like, behavioral in nature. A physical cue is something that will happen on its own – breathing, heartbeat, eye twitch. Conversely, behavioral cues are learned behaviors that are connected to emotions. Pacing, gritting your teeth, wringing your hands, and talking to yourself are all behavioral cues. Like all the other cues listed above, behavioral cues are things that happen without conscious thought, yet they are activities that we can be aware of and stop.

Homework

Craving Levels:

S ___ M ___ T ___ W ___ T ___ F ___ S ___

Situation/Event: (situations or events that lead to a desire to use/drink)

1. ____________________
2. ____________________
3. ____________________
4. ____________________
5. ____________________

Feelings/Thoughts: (emotions or thoughts that lead to a desire to use/drink)

1. ____________________
2. ____________________
3. ____________________
4. ____________________
5. ____________________

Cues: (mental/physical/behavioral cues that accompany or precede a desire to use/drink)

1. ____________________
2. ____________________
3. ____________________
4. ____________________
5. ____________________

Urges: (thoughts or self-talk that create urges or cravings to use/drink)

1. ____________________
2. ____________________
3. ____________________
4. ____________________
5. ____________________

The Recovery Battle

SESSION 6:

Recovery Battle

We all fight many battles in our lives. Those enemies and the outcome of those conflicts shape addiction, recovery, and relapse. In these battles we all have allies and tools that protect and help us on the battlefield of recovery. This exercise is designed to help you remove yourself from the real world battle which can make looking at the entire scene difficult. Instead of simply listing the objects that stand in the way or the items and people who assist us, in this worksheet we put it in the context of a medieval, fantasy-style battle.

<u>Opponents to recovery</u>

The most obvious opponent in this battle is your metaphorical dragon.. Most commonly, there is one large obstacle that impacts recovery. A dragon can be any number of things – people, places, events, all which have a massive impact on addiction, recovery, and relapse. The dragon's flame represents the items that weaken your recovery.. And while the dragon is the biggest opponent to sustained recovery, there are also soldiers who battle alongside the dragon. This opposing force is made up of the smaller items that alone may or may not lead to relapse or continued use. Yet when there is more than one solider present, they can overpower you and also seem stronger when the dragon is there.

<u>Allies to recovery</u>

When attempting recovery, remember there are those people, places, and things that help empower and protect your recovery, as well. The shield represents those things that serve to protect your recovery. These can be activities, places, even faith and beliefs. Our greatest allies are often those who stand behind us and help us stand tall when we are weak. Don't confuse these allies with the idea that we are not the hero of the story. These allies are those who support us, but we are the ones who must be willing to fight the battle and sound the horn to charge ahead on the battlefield, leading the troops to victory in recovery.

Homework

Craving Levels:

S ___ M ___ T ___ W ___ T ___ F ___ S ___

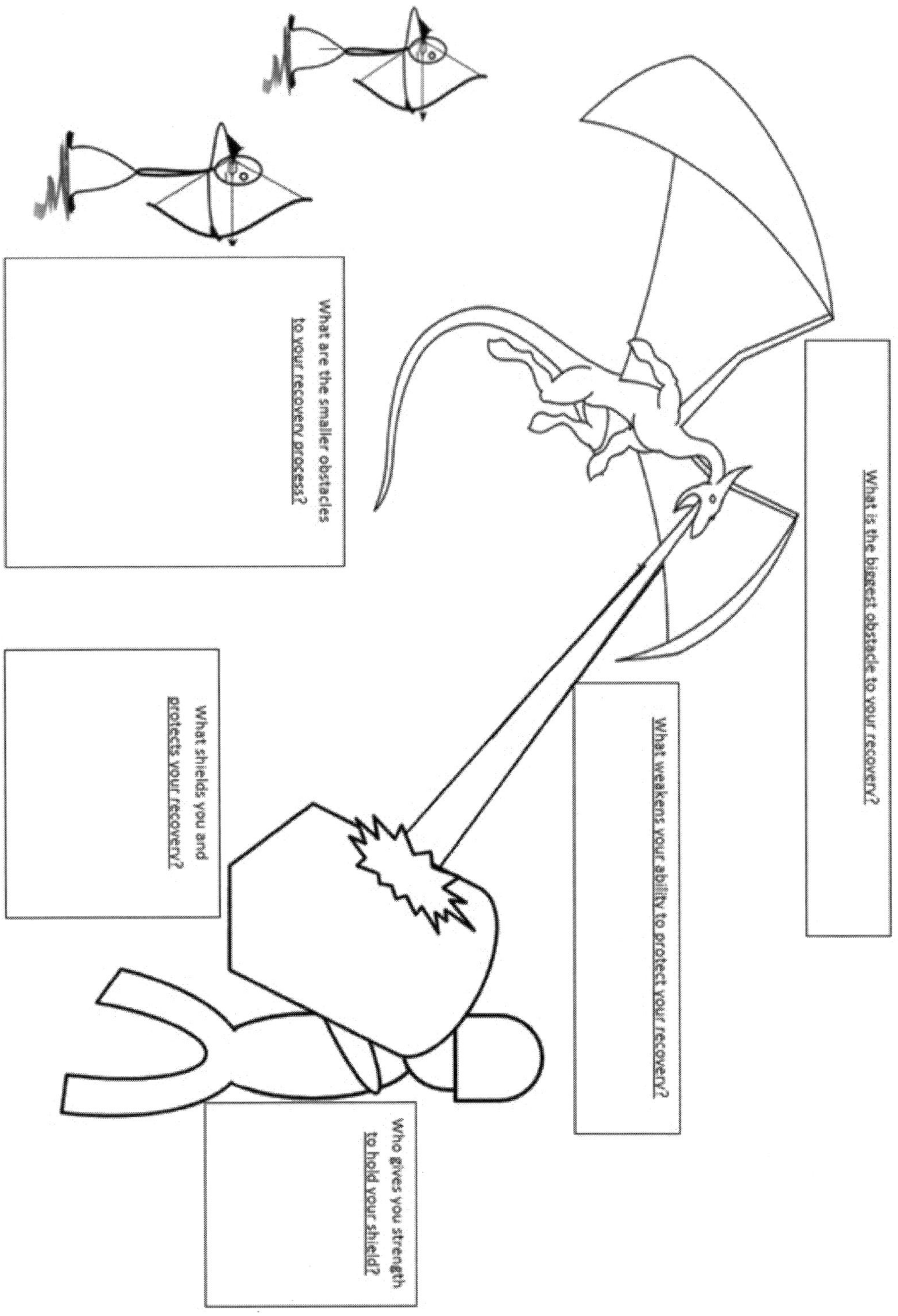

Event Assessments

SESSION 7:

Learning to Assess Events

As previously discussed, events are things which happen that are often outside our control. Yet, by changing the people, places, and things with which we spend our time, we can limit these events. This may be a set feature, but it is the whole of what we are analyzing, so choose events which may be difficult and have created a desire to use or may impact your recovery. What happened? What was the first event that led to those urges or cravings? What started you down that path; was it a break up, being late to work, getting fired, or a celebration with friends?

Emotional thoughts are based on how we feel. They lack logic for that reason, and their creation often occurs without conscious thought, but happens more in our gut.

Facts are much like the event: they are items that cannot be disputed, except by allowing emotions to interfere with our thought processes and therefore make us have those emotional thoughts which are skewed. It is out of the facts that logical thoughts are developed; these are the thoughts about what may be the reason for an event, if we remove our emotional thoughts and are able to step back from the situation. By pulling facts out of the event and looking at them, we also better understand our vulnerabilities, which are the items that when added to the event create our emotional thoughts.

When you combine the facts of the event and vulnerabilities, we create our perception about the event. This is different than our reality, but is a key piece of what creates our reality. Our perception, when combined with logical and emotional thoughts, is what creates our reality. Our reality is what we believe to be true, not true facts, but facts impacted by our insecurities.

What is reality? Reality is our worldview. It is a combination of all the items; it is what we believe to be true when we add each of the other pieces together. Our reality is not wrong, but it can and, at times, must be shifted and this happens not always due to a desire to change, but because of every experience we have. Every experience includes all the items in this event assessment, and the outcome is the shifting or reinforcement of our reality.

Homework

Craving Levels:

S ___ M ___ T ___ W ___ T ___ F ___ S ___

Event: ______________________________

____

____

____

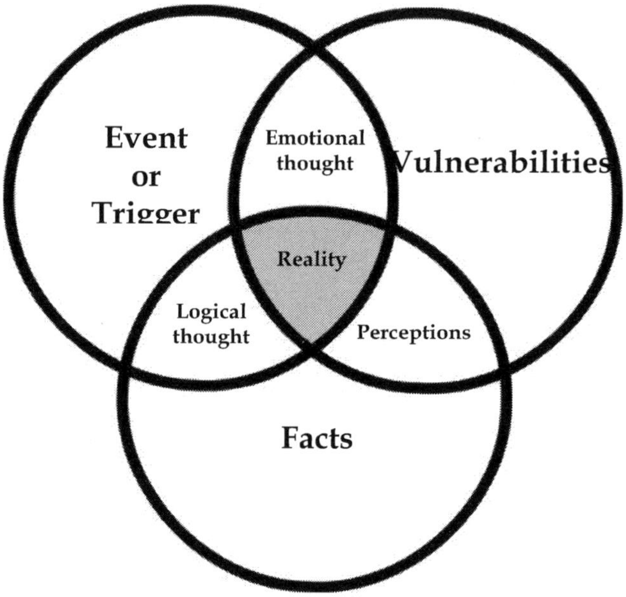

Vulnerabilities: ______________________________

____

____

____

Emotional thoughts: ______________________________

____

____

Facts: ______________________________

____

____

Logical thoughts: ______________________________

____

____

Reality: ______________________________

____

____

Change Plans

SESSION 8:

Creating a Plan for Change

Creating active change such as recovery is accomplished not by chance, but by setting a clear goal. Once a goal is set, in this case recovery, then the work can begin. Any active change or goal is motivated by something; there are feelings and beliefs which make that change something we desire to create. Behind that motivation are the values which drive that motivation and desire to create change. Values for some may be family or God, but for others, they may be completely different. When it comes to motivation, the danger is that some people desire to change on the idea that it will return things to how they were before. It the desired outcome is not achieved, it can create a dangerous trigger for relapse.

With any goal as large as recovery and preventing relapse, there are steps involved in reaching the goal. Smaller goals or items must be completed before the large goal itself can be accomplished. With these smaller steps, setting a timeline is important to know if the plan for change is working.

One must understand both the people and things that can help with reaching the goal and also those people and items that may prevent reaching the goal. This can be hard to look at since it may mean removing people, places, and things from our lives, ones we may feel we want to remain.

Just as with the timeline, the smaller steps need to be measurable, and there must be an understanding of how to measure whether they are being accomplished or not. If the goals are not being reached, knowing what to do is important. Often this means revisiting the smaller steps. Perhaps they are too large or perhaps they are items once believed to help, but now must be changed or adjusted so to help with recovery and preventing relapse. When or if this occurs, it can mean the creation of an entirely new change plan, addition of supplemental steps, or adjustment to existing steps towards that goal.

If relapse occurs, this does not necessarily mean that the change plan is incorrect, but instead, that it may need adjustment. The issue could possibly be not staying true to the change plan, so an honest assessment of the steps and if they were being taken is necessary. This means reviewing the plan – the steps, helpful and harmful people and items, and the way measuring the plan is being done.

Homework

Craving Levels:

S ___ M ___ T ___ W ___ T ___ F ___ S ___

What goal do you want to reach? What change do you want to create?
What is the motivation for this goal?
What value is driving this motivation or goal?
What steps will it take to reach this goal?
What is your timeline for reaching this goal?
What are the things that will help you reach this goal?

Who are the people who can help you reach this goal?
What are the things that can interfere with this goal?
Who are the people who can interfere with this goal?
How will you measure if your plan is working?
What will you do if this plan isn't working?

Responsive vs. Reactive

SESSION 9:

Internal Stairs: Responsive vs. Reactive

Our internal messages can cloud our ability to see things for what they truly are. The major difference between being reactive and being responsive is the difference between letting emotions and the event control the situation or taking control of the situation and allowing logic to assist with being responsive to prevent the negative outcomes such as relapse.

The key is to look at each of these pieces individually. We have discussed understanding our vulnerabilities and other factors that create our reality and worldview. This is where this exercise, like others, begins because this is where we exist. The event or trigger is viewed as that item which may cause you to stumble in your recovery. It is the item you will encounter in recovery which has the potential to cause relapse or strengthen your recovery.

First, look at the possible negative consequences. These happen when a person is reactive to a situation rather than responsive. When the event happens, what has been the course that has happened in the past that led to deeper and larger issues? As you go down the stairs, you are damaged, and you damage others more and more. Each step down is the next item in the chain of events.

Next, look at the responsive side, when you allow the event and emotions alone to control the situation. Rather than falling down the stairs, you climb to a better outcome. Similar to the reactive side, in the responsive piece, look at how a positive chain of events would occur. When looking at this, you can break down the responsive interaction to see how each step leads to climbing to the next, and how you gain greater height and strength as a result of the other. This understanding serves to strengthen the resolve to be responsive as you understand the positive end result that can occur when you don't allow the situation and emotions to control what follows the event.

Responsive vs Reactive: Internal Stairs Worksheet

Our internal messages can cloud our ability to see things for what they truly are. When we are aware of our vulnerabilities and the internal messages we carry within us we can see the triggers and obstacles to using logical thought. When we see things logically and are able to climb the steps to successful emotional and logic pairing instead of falling down the path to chaos

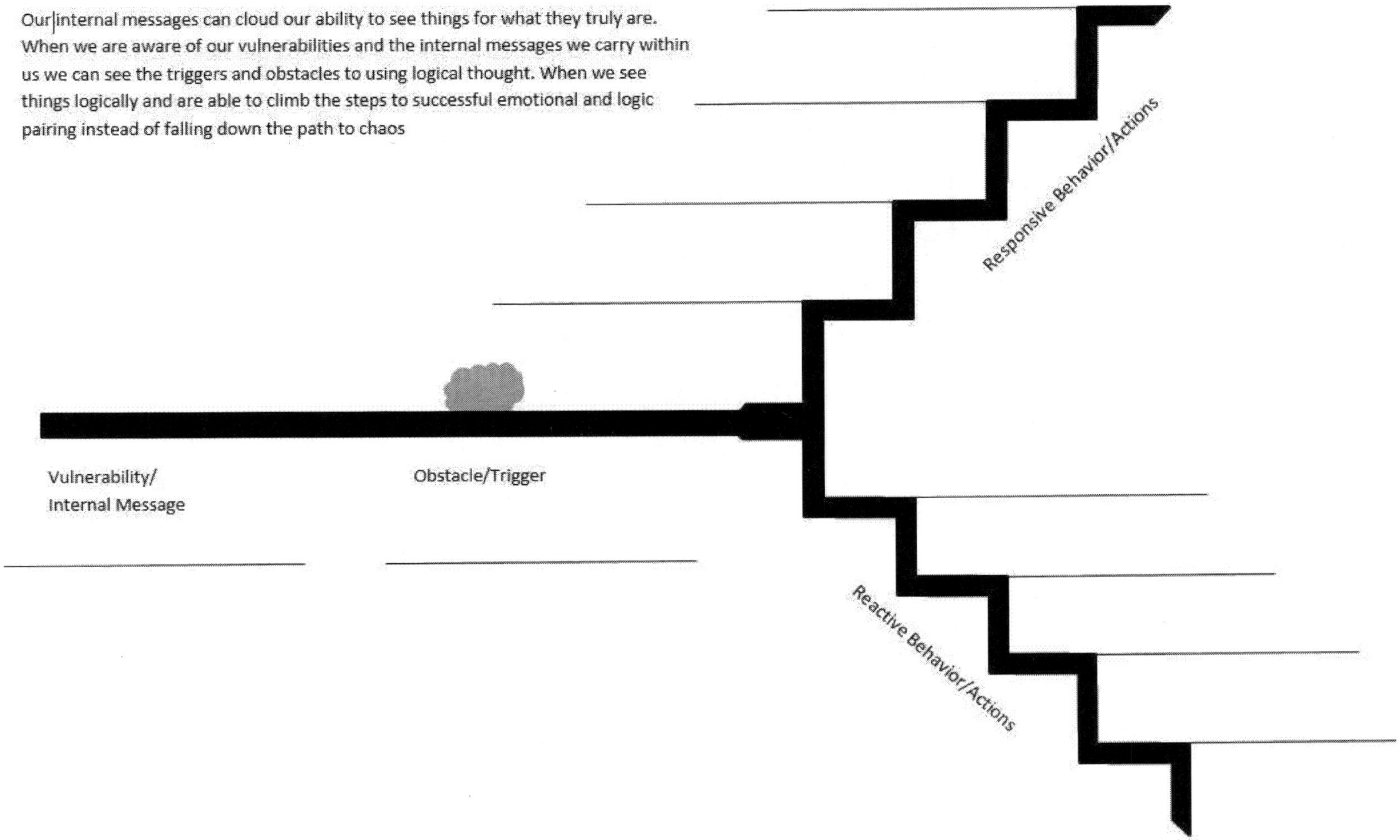

Homework

Craving Levels:

S ___ M ___ T ___ W ___ T ___ F ___ S ___

Ashamed of Shame

SESSION 10:

People often mistake shame and being ashamed as the same thing, but they are very different from a clinical standpoint. Being ashamed is a moment-to-moment event; shame is something that is carried long term. An easier way to explain it might be to say being ashamed is *"I did something bad"* while shame is *"I am bad."* As such, shame and being ashamed impact a person in drastically different ways.

The interesting part of shame is that it is us labeling ourselves and developing inner messages that influence every interaction we have. So long as we believe those shame words and phrases are true, we will continue to limit ourselves and give the past power over the present and future. To address shame, it must be broken down and combatted as inaccurate; for shame is almost without fail statements that are false, but we tell ourselves they are true.

To break down and combat the shame words and phrases we hold, it takes looking at the times when you are negative about yourself. Do you say "I did something stupid" or "I am stupid"? The first is being ashamed; the second is shame, and most likely it is something that you tell yourself repeatedly. Those are the negative items you are looking for that you tell yourself over and over.

Once you identify the words and phrases to which your shame is connected, you must also consider when you feel that way. When do you feel stupid? When do you feel worthless? Next, think about who in your past has said these words or phrases to you. Most often, the shame words are created by people that on some level we respect: a parent, a teacher, a coach, a past lover. If it was someone who didn't matter to us, then the words would not have the power they do. While others plant the seeds of shame, we are the ones who must stop watering them.

After breaking down the shame words and phrases, combatting it is a matter of realizing that shame words are very black and white, but they all have exceptions to them. Are you always stupid? Most likely not, but that is what we tell ourselves in the moments when the shame words surface.

After you list your shame words, list the opposite of that word, and then ask yourself if there are times that the opposite is true. If your shame word, for example, is "worthless", the opposite would be "value". What are the times and things that you have that you value? If you have a pet, a child, or a skill that serves a purpose, you have some value. If you have some value that combats the idea you are worthless, worthless is without value.

Homework

Craving Levels:

S ___ M ___ T ___ W ___ T ___ F ___ S ___

Shame Word	When Felt	Who Has Said

Shame Word/Phrase	Opposite	When Felt

What We Tell Ourselves

SESSION 11:

The Story That Shame Wrote

If shame is the seed we have allowed others to plant and which we have continued to water, our internal message would be the root system of the entire forest. It is the large mat that allows all interactions in the forest, but it is also something that we rarely see or even contemplate. Understanding our shame allows us to look deeper at our internal message and how what we tell ourselves impacts every interaction we have.

Each person has his or her own experiences and internal message that has been created, reinforced, and transformed from a passing thought to a concrete reality. How do we explore our story so we can rewrite it? Naming and letting go. We give power to words, and we let them have power over our thoughts. We all name the events that we experience. "Another bad day," "it's a crisis," or "wonderful weekend" are all examples of naming. Some are positive, and some are negative.

Once we have named an event or situation, we have given up some of the power, but when we let go, we take back that power we have given to a situation. Part of life is letting go – of plans, dreams, and even people. It is only by letting go of these items and ideas that we can move on through life, but part of letting go is understanding why we hold on and why we must let go.

<u>Homework</u>

Craving Levels:

S ___ M ___ T ___ W ___ T ___ F ___ S ___

The only thing we truly have the ability to control is our response to a given situation. The key to changing how we react when something happens is to change our own internal self-talk from negative to positive. The way we do this is by understanding what we are feeling, why we are feeling it, and letting go of the negative to support ourselves.

NAMING:
We all name the events that we experience. "Another bad day," "it's a crisis," or "wonderful weekend" are all examples of naming. Some are positive, and some are negative.

Choose a recent event:____
How did you name it at the time:____
What is a positive/negative name you could give it:____
If that event happened to a friend, what would you name it:___________________________________
Do you think reframing the event would have changed your response:_____________________________
Explain why/why not:____

LETTING GO:

Part of life is letting go – of plans, dreams, and even people. It is only by letting go of these items and ideas that we can move on through life, but part of letting go is understanding why we hold on and why we must let go.

Choose three items/ideas/people you need to let go:____

____

If those things or people were out of your life, what emotions would you have about it?
1. ____
2. ____
3. ____

If you have negative emotions about them being gone, is there a positive emotion as well?___________
If yes, explain:____
What advice would you give about these items or feelings to a friend?____

INTERNAL MESSAGE:

We each have internal messages that we tell ourselves, sometimes without even realizing we do this. These messages can be supportive, but can also tear us down.

Sit quietly and close your eyes. What negative things are you telling yourself?_____________________

____

What negative messages do you often hear?____

____

Write the positive message that is the opposite of them:______________________________________

____

How would things change if you were telling yourself the positive?____

Shame and Unlocking the Box

SESSION 12:

The Pandora's Box of Our Mind

Zeus gave a box as a wedding present to Pandora and Epimetheus. The box was locked, and it had come with a note which read "DO NOT OPEN." Attached to the note, however, was the key to the box. Pandora knew she should not open the box, but one day her curiosity got the better of her, and she unlocked the box and opened it. When the lid was raised, out flew all of the bad things which now exist in the world: envy, sickness, hate, disease. Pandora slammed the lid closed, but it was too late, and she began to weep.

As Pandora wept, Epimetheus heard her and came running to where she sat. Pandora opened the lid to show her husband the box was empty. When she opened the lid a tiny bug flew out. The bug smiled at Pandora, a thank you for freedom, before flying away. The tiny bug was Hope, and hope made all the difference in the world.

By opening the box, Pandora exposed herself and the rest of the world to hurt and evil, but without opening the box, hope never would have been released into the world. Just like in Pandora's case, we must expose ourselves to the hurt that we hold within. For as long as we keep the hurt locked away, so too do we lock away hope.

The way we unlock the box is far different than Pandora's case as no one has provided us a key, but it is by telling our story that we are able to understand more and more what our internal message is and how we can find our own hope. Again, unlike Pandora, what we find when we open the box is different. We find little hurt, little evils, and a little hope, but also another box. When telling your story to another, you may hold back items, but write the story knowing no one will see it. No matter who you have hurt, what you have done, or who has hurt you, tell the whole story.

Homework

Craving Levels:

S ___ M ___ T ___ W ___ T ___ F ___ S ___

My Story:

Reframing the Story

SESSION 13:

Write a New Meaning to Your Story

Unlike an author who can rewrite an entire story, in life we can only change how the chapters left to write turn out. In those chapters, we are able to give new meaning to the prior chapters. Just like in great novels, what started as sad stories filled with hurt which then motivate the hero in the second half of the book, this too can be what all the events that occurred during relapse or active using can become. We can't delete the story from before recovery, but it can be the driving force for life once it is reframed as motivation.

Think about those past events as you work through the worksheet. What is the unhealthy way you have viewed the event? Think about how you would talk about that thought with a friend or family member, the things which show that thought isn't reality. Reframe those thoughts as motivation rather than a reason to punish yourself.

Example:

Perhaps you cheated on your spouse when actively using and that led to divorce. Most would consider that event as something you wished never happened and would be angry over it because that hurt can never go away. The contradiction is that the hurt can go away. That event probably led to the choice to stop using and seek treatment or was a motivation in recovery. Most would also likely tell a friend or family member not to punish him or herself for something he or she can't change. The healthy thought would be that while it was not the right thing to do, out of that hurt came a lot of positive outcomes, and if you are to marry again, you will most likely be that much more dedicated of a partner.

Homework

Craving Levels:

S ___ M ___ T ___ W ___ T ___ F ___ S ___

Unhealthy/Unhelpful Thought:
Is there evidence that contradicts? **Are there exceptions where this thought is untrue?** **Is there a pattern of these thoughts?** **What would you say if a friend thought this?** **Is there a different way to think about this?**
Healthy/Fact Based Thought:

Relapse Prevention Plan

SESSION 14:

Preventing Relapse

Having worked through this program, you have gained a greater understanding of what emotional and physical items have impacted how you feel about yourself and have gained an understanding of your addiction. Recovery is a daily practice, and one of the best ways to protect that recovery on a daily basis is to have a relapse prevention plan.

As you complete the relapse prevention plan below, you will find items that connect to all the aspects discussed over the course of this group. Every group, every exercise, all of your work to this point has been preparing you not to complete this plan, but to go out into life and manage and protect your recovery.

Look at the events that led to using and that may have led to relapse previously. These are some situations which may be triggers in the future, as well. Additionally, consider the emotions you felt when the event occurred, or the emotions which have led to use or relapse, regardless of the event or situation. Continue to the thoughts you had, your perceptions, your reality, your self-talk.

Look at the positives of not relapsing and the possible negative impact of using. Three of the most important questions related to your continued recovery are: who can you talk to, what else can you do, and what are the emotional outcomes of continued recovery. The first two questions help remind you who your supports are. None of us are alone; yet different situations may require us to talk to different people. Activities that help stop thoughts of relapse or alleviate stress before the thoughts of relapse happen are supports we do for ourselves, but again, different situations mean different activities. The last question, *what is the emotional outcome of continued recovery*, relates to those values, that motivation that led to change and a reminder of the need to protect your recovery in good times but especially in not so good times.

Homework

Craving Levels:

S ___ M ___ T ___ W ___ T ___ F ___ S ___

Where were you? What were you doing?	
What emotions were you feeling? How intense (1-10)?	
What were your negative thoughts?	
What are the outcomes of relapse? 1. 2. 3. 4. 5.	**What are the outcomes of not using?** 1. 2. 3. 4. 5.
What can you do instead of drinking/using?	
Who can you talk to about the situation?	
What is the emotional outcome of continued recovery?	

Made in the USA
Monee, IL
08 November 2026

68144953R00022